Core Exercises for Seniors Over 60

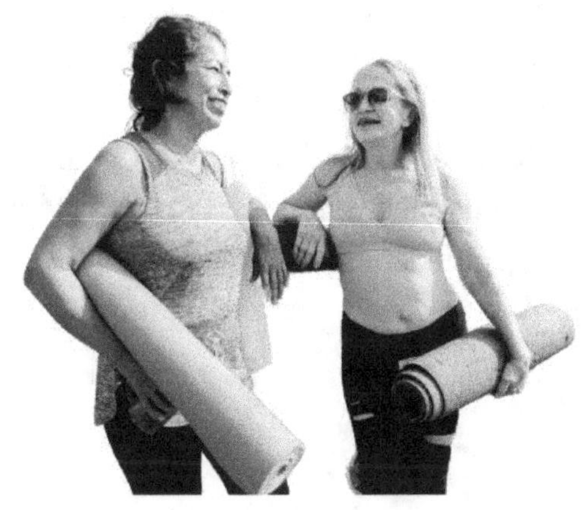

A Comprehensive Guide to Build Balance and Boost Strength, Energy and Confidence

Stacey R. Smith

Table of Content

Introduction

Reclaim Your Strength and Independence: Why Core Exercises Matter After 60

Dispelling Myths and Building Confidence: Understanding Your Unique Body

Setting Realistic Goals and Finding Joy in Movement

Creating Your Blueprint

Benefits of Core Exercises for Seniors

Chapter 1: Building a Strong Core

Uncovering the Mysteries of Magic

Putting Together Your Powerhouse

Unleash Your Potential

Bonus Suggestions

When to Exercise

Pay Attention to Your Inner DJ

Where to Exercise

Identifying Your Oasis

Proper Breathing Techniques

More Than Just Motion

Chapter 2: Seated Core Exercises

Chapter 3: Standing Core Exercises

Chapter 4: Mat Core Exercises

Chapter 5: Walking Core Exercises

Chapter 6: Partners Exercises

Chapter 7: Exercises with Weights

Chapter 8: Exercises for Ache and Pain Relieve

Chapter 9: Nutrition Tips for Core Health
Importance of a Balanced Diet
Foods that Support Core Strength
Conclusion
Workout Planner

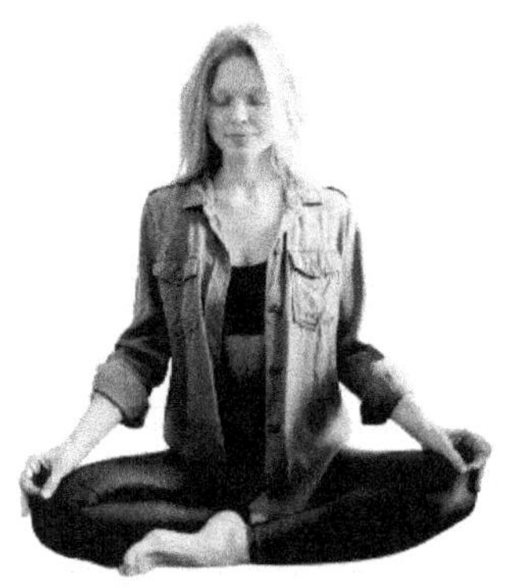

Introduction

The morning fog lingered over the park, matching Margaret's anxiety. Balance wasn't what it used to be at 62. Gardening, which had previously been a delight, now bore the threat of shaky ankles and shattered pride. "Getting older is no picnic," she groaned as she handed me a warm mug of tea.

Then I told her about my new book, "Core Exercises for Seniors Over 60." She flicked over the pages hesitantly, attracted by the soft stances and encouraging phrases. "March in Place?" she said with a grin, "Maybe 'Side plank' is more my style."

But then something happened. She was drawn in by the promise of recovered strength, greater flexibility, and even a hint of rebellion against age. We began with basic stretches by the window, her laughing covering her hand tremors. Slowly, the park called once more. As she performed "Mat Core Exercises" on the dewy grass, bird singing replaced her apprehension, and the light warmed her grin.

Days progressed into weeks, and the formerly timid motions gained confidence. Balance reappeared, like a long-forgotten tune. Gardening became a dance for her, her motions sure and forceful. As she reached for sun-drenched flowers, the book became her friend, its wisdom whispered on the breeze.

I spotted her by the lake one morning, giggling as she casually touched her toes. "Look!" she said, her eyes sparkling like dew in the morning. "The book wasn't just about exercises, it was about rediscovering myself."

Margaret's tale isn't unique to her. It's a witness to the transforming power of "Core Exercises for Seniors Over 60," the power of movement, the tenacity of the soul, and the transformative magic of "Core Exercises for Seniors Over 60." It's the kind of book that says, "It's not too late," then demonstrates it, one small step at a time.

So, take a risk. Open the book, accept the possibilities, and rediscover the inner strength, balance, and, yes, joy. Every bend, every stretch is a victory song, a reminder that the dance floor of life embraces us all, regardless of age.

Begin your trip right now. Allow "Core Exercises for Seniors Over 60" to guide you to your own sun-drenched success beside the lake.

Reclaim Your Strength and Independence: Why Core Exercises Matter After 60

Turning 60 does not have to mean resignation to infirmity. Our bodies may alter as we age, but within us is a secret strength waiting to be ignited - the power of a strong core. Forget six-pack abs; the true magic of core workouts for seniors is restoring strength, freedom, and the vivid tapestry of everyday life.

Imagine waking up without the grumble of tight joints, gardening without the worry of unsteady ankles, or simply rising from a chair with grace. These are the benefits of having a strong core. It's not only about vanity; it's about restoring your independence and confidence.

Consider your core to be the powerhouse of your body. It's the unseen symphony director, orchestrating every action, from walking and climbing stairs to carrying groceries and smiling with your grandkids. A strong core is more than simply sculpted abs; it also means better balance and stability, better posture, and even sharper cognitive performance. It's the cornerstone for all of your everyday activities, the silent protector against falls and injuries.

But, let's face it, age can impair this critical area. Years of sitting at a desk, repetitive strain, or chronic discomfort can cause our core muscles to be neglected, depriving us of our young mobility. This does not have to be our fate. "Core Exercises for Seniors Over 60" is a gentle yet effective approach to strengthening your core from the ground up.

Forget about daunting gym programs and lengthy crunches. Our book takes a personalized approach to core training, with exercises for beginners that you can practice anywhere, at any time. Consider chair-based workouts that revitalize your muscles without requiring you to leave your seat, or easy stretches that awaken your core while you enjoy the morning light.

This isn't simply about exercising; it's about rediscovering oneself. You'll learn how to incorporate activity into your everyday routine, discover joy in the process, and stay motivated throughout your journey. With each bend and stretch, you'll feel a revitalized feeling of strength, a greater confidence in your body, and the freedom to recover your independence.

Turning 60 isn't a death sentence; it's an invitation to discover hidden strengths. "Core Exercises for Seniors Over 60" is your guide, your friend on your quest to regain your vibrant self. Accept the possibilities, open the book, and restore your strength one gentle workout at a time.

Join the movement. It is never too late to be powerful, independent, and fully alive.

Dispelling Myths and Building Confidence: Understanding Your Unique Body

Aging is a tapestry of experiences intertwined with knowledge, humor, and maybe a fair amount of cynicism. Myths and misunderstandings abound when it comes to fitness, particularly core workouts, making many seniors afraid to begin on a road to a stronger self. Let's dispel these myths and boost your confidence by learning about your unique physique at 60 and beyond.

Myth #1: You're "too old" to begin: Nonsense! Age is merely a number, and your body is capable of tremendous adaptation and rejuvenation. You may nurture inner strength and core stability at every stage of life, just as a seasoned gardener does with a variety plot.

Myth #2: Core exercises are all about getting six-pack abs: Forget crunches if you want sculpted abs! A solid core for seniors is about much more than looks. It's about having better posture, better balance, and the freedom to go about your daily life with confidence. Consider reaching for a high shelf, bending to tie your shoes, or receiving a hug from a grandchild without worry of back discomfort.

Myth #3: You need expensive equipment or a gym membership to exercise: Forget about high-priced electronics and frightening crowds. Your body is your ultimate gym, and "Core Exercises for Seniors Over 60" equips you to work out wherever and whenever you want. Your chair converts into a launchpad for core-activating stretches, your living room floor into a moderate yoga class, and the park into a natural balancing playground.

Myth #4: It's excruciatingly unpleasant and monotonous: Exercise does not have to be a chore! "Core Exercises for Seniors Over 60" focuses on low-impact, gentle exercises that are suited to your unique requirements and limitations. You'll discover the pleasure of mindful stretches that wake up your core and leave you feeling energized rather than weary.

Building Confidence Through Understanding

Understanding your individual physique is essential for developing confidence. Pay attention to your body's whispers, accept its limitations, and rejoice in its accomplishments. Accept changes and adjustments, recognizing that little, steady actions lead to significant changes.

"Core Exercises for Seniors Over 60" is your traveling companion on your adventure. We recognize the aches and frustrations of aging, yet we provide compassionate treatments and empowering guidance. You'll learn to read your body's language, recognize pain causes, and avoid injury while pushing your limits in a supportive and safe atmosphere.

Keep in mind that you are not alone. Core workouts are helping millions of seniors regain their power and independence. With each bend and stretch, you will gain confidence in your body, unearth its hidden capabilities, and demonstrate to yourself that strength and flexibility have no age limit.

So, let go of the misconceptions, enjoy the adventure, and let "Core Exercises for Seniors Over 60" lead you to a stronger, more confident self. It's time to rewrite your own story, one step at a time!

Setting Realistic Goals and Finding Joy in Movement

Turning 60 does not have to be the end of your fitness goals. It's only a simple recalibration, a shift away from chasing impossible ideals and toward setting doable objectives and discovering the surprising delight in movement. Imagine waking up not fearful of the "must-dos," but excited about the "can-dos" your strengthened core will enable.

Forget about crash diets and punishing workouts. "Core Exercises for Seniors Over 60" suggests a gentler, more long-term approach. We believe in recognizing minor accomplishments and creating realistic objectives for your individual body and lifestyle. Consider ascending the stairs without puffing, strolling around the park with renewed vigor, or just leaning down to tie your shoes without a grimace. These, not Olympic accomplishments, are the ultimate indicators of senior fitness success.

But how can we get motivation in "realistic" situations? The solution is to rediscover the basic joy of movement. Forget the tedium of "should-dos" and embrace the vivacious dance of "can-dos."

Consider the sun-kissed pleasure of a slow morning stretch, the energizing rhythm of chair-based core exercises, or the freeing flow of a stroll through the park. Motivation arises organically when activity becomes a celebration of what your body can achieve rather than a punishment for what it cannot.

Creating Your Blueprint

1. Begin Small, But Dream Big: Begin with small, attainable objectives, such as climbing a flight of stairs without stopping or holding a plank for 30 seconds. As you overcome these, your confidence will skyrocket, driving you to larger goals.

2. Listen to your Body: Respect your limits and appreciate your talents by listening to your body. Learn to tell the difference between a healthy challenge and a possible injury. Modify exercises as required to create a tailored symphony of movement in your core regimen.

3. Accept "movement snacks": Forget about long, arduous exercises. Divide your daily routine into bite-sized "movement snacks" of five minutes here and ten minutes there. This method keeps you engaged, stimulated, and motivated.

4. Find your Joy: Discover activities that fire your enthusiasm for movement, whether it's dancing to your favorite tunes, doing yoga in the garden, or swimming laps at the neighborhood pool. When you're having fun, you never feel compelled.

Benefits of Core Exercises for Seniors

As elders gracefully traverse their golden years, preserving excellent health becomes a top priority. Core strength is a cornerstone of well-being that frequently takes center stage, and engaging in deliberate core exercises brings forth a slew of advantages that are specifically geared to the requirements of those over 60.

1. Improved Stability and Balance:

Strengthening core muscles improves stability, lowers the chance of falling, and improves general balance. This is especially important for elderly who want to keep their independence and avoid mishaps.

2. Improved Posture:

Core workouts help to improve posture by supporting the spine. Seniors have better alignment, which reduces the probability of developing musculoskeletal problems related to bad posture.

3. Mobility and joint health:

Core workouts encourage optimal body mechanics, reducing joint tension. This is advantageous for seniors, particularly those suffering from illnesses such as arthritis, since it may lead to improved joint health and enhanced mobility.

4. Fitness for Function:

Core strength makes it simpler to do daily tasks like bending, reaching, and lifting. Seniors find these jobs easier to complete, supporting independence and an active lifestyle.

5. Reduced Back Pain in the Lower Back:

Many seniors suffer from lower back pain, and focused core workouts are a natural and efficient way to relieve discomfort. Strengthening the core muscles helps to stabilize the spine and relieves lower back discomfort.

6. The Mind-Body Connection:

Core exercises need concentration and focus, building a strong mind-body connection. This mindfulness factor not only improves the efficiency of the workouts, but it also helps with stress reduction and mental well-being.

7. Gained Functional Independence:

A strong core leads to greater functional independence. Seniors are more competent to execute everyday duties without the aid of others, fostering a sense of self-sufficiency.

8. Influence on Cardiovascular Health:

Some active core workouts can raise the heart rate, which benefits cardiovascular health. While not a substitute for regular cardiovascular exercise, integrating these factors improves overall fitness.

9. Respiratory Function Improvement:

Controlled breathing patterns are frequently used in core workouts. This not only improves respiratory function but also highlights the necessity of attentive breathing, which has broader health implications.

10. Improved Digestive Health:

Certain core exercises can activate abdominal muscles and help with digestion. While not a direct replacement for a good diet, these workouts can help with general digestive health.

Essentially, the advantages of core workouts for seniors go much beyond physical strength. They embody a comprehensive approach to well-being, allowing people to enjoy the richness of life with vigor and confidence.

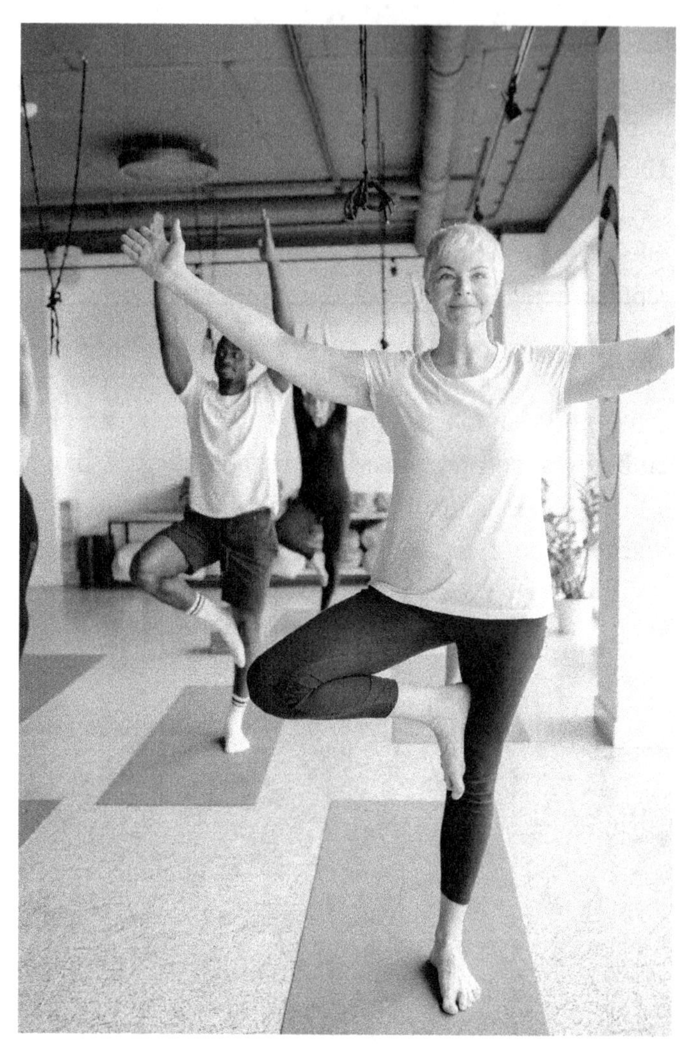

15|Core Exercises for Seniors Over 60

Chapter 1: Building a Strong Core

Forget about six-pack fantasies and gym-bunny ambitions. Building a strong core after the age of 60 is about far more than looks; it's about reclaiming a lively, independent life. It's about taking the stairs without gasping, stooping to tie your shoes without suffering, and embracing ordinary activities with renewed zeal.

Consider your core to be your body's hidden orchestra conductor. It's not just your abs, but they're important. It's a symphony of stomach, back, and side muscles that work together to offer stability, posture, and support for every action you make. Consider it your body's internal corset, keeping everything in place while allowing you to move with strength and accuracy.

However, aging has its drawbacks. Muscle mass inevitably falls, and our core is often one of the first to suffer. This can cause a chain reaction of problems, ranging from back discomfort and bad posture to impaired balance and an increased chance of falling.

It's never too late to restore and strengthen your core! "Core Exercises for Seniors Over 60" provides a safe, gentle, and effective method for reawakening this dormant powerhouse.

Uncovering the Mysteries of Magic

1. Beyond the Six-Pack: Forget crunches if you want sculpted abs! Our emphasis is on functional strength and stability, which will help you in your daily life.

2. The Invisible Designer: Learn how a strong core benefits not only your physical health (balance, posture, pain reduction), but also your mental health (cognitive function, mood enhancement).

3. Busting Myths: There will be no grueling gym routines or expensive equipment. We provide simple, low-impact workouts that you may do anywhere, at any time.

Putting Together Your Powerhouse

1. First and foremost, master the fundamentals of posture and alignment to establish a firm foundation for your core workouts.

2. Begin with easy movements that activate your core without effort, gradually increasing strength and confidence.

3. Not Perfection, but Progression. Modify workouts as required, listen to your body, and appreciate tiny accomplishments. The key is progress, not perfection.

4. Breathe, imagine, and connect with your movements to strengthen your mind-body

connection. Engage your thoughts to get the most out of your workouts.

Unleash Your Potential

As you strengthen your core, you will notice a physical, mental, and emotional shift. You will benefit from:

1. Improved Balance and Stability: Forget about falling and shaky ankles. A strong core keeps you balanced and on your feet.

2. Posture Improvement: Stand tall and confident! Say goodbye to bent shoulders and back ache by discovering the elegance and relaxation that comes with proper posture.

3. Greater Movement Ease: Bending, lifting, and reaching become second nature as your core muscles operate in unison.

4. Increased Energy and Vitality: Feel the energizing force of movement! A strong core energizes your body and improves your attitude.

5. Emotional Boost: Celebrate your tiny and huge accomplishments! Developing your core is a path of self-awareness and empowerment.

"Core Exercises for Seniors Over 60" is your roadmap for power, stability, and independence. It's not only about workouts; it's about discovering your hidden potential. Accept the journey, appreciate your accomplishments, and rediscover the joy of exercise. Remember, aging is not a death sentence;

it is an opportunity to rediscover the power you never knew you possessed. Begin your path today, and watch your core become the maestro of a dynamic, self-sufficient existence after the age of 60.

Bonus Suggestions

1. Find a fun activity that involves core strengthening, such as dance, yoga, or swimming.
2. Include movement in your daily routine by using the stairs, doing exercises while watching TV, or gardening in attentive postures.
3. Keep hydrated! Water is necessary for muscular function as well as general health.
4. Track your progress and celebrate your accomplishments, it will keep you motivated and on track.
5. Join a community, locate a workout companion or a senior fitness club for motivation and support.
Building a solid foundation is an investment in your future. It's about rediscovering your inner power, freedom, and the vivid tapestry of daily life. Take the first step now and allow your core to guide you to a more powerful, happy, and empowered self.

When to Exercise

The alarm goes off, the daylight snoozes through the blinds, and the age-old question: when should I exercise? Morning fighters are those who wake with the lark, while midnight owls swear by moonlit exercises. The fact is that the "perfect" hour is more about listening to your body and finding synergy with your lifestyle than it is about the clock.

1. Morning Songs:

For some, daybreak is the ideal time to workout. Cortisol, the body's natural energy enhancer, rises in the morning, providing you a competitive advantage. Morning workouts can help raise your metabolism, increase your attention throughout the day, and provide a sense of achievement before the daily grind begins. Plus, around morning, the gym is generally less busy!

2. Momentum at Midday:

Lunchtime workouts can provide a nice reprieve from the monotony of the workweek. A sweat session in the middle of the day can increase alertness, reduce tension, and even boost creativity for your afternoon duties. Just be sure to leave enough time to change, shower, and refuel before returning to work.

3. Evening Reminiscences:

The gym after dark is a haven for night owls. Evening workouts may be a terrific way to unwind after a long day, increase sleep quality (if scheduled correctly), and provide a feeling of closure before bed. However, late-night workouts that stimulate your nervous system too close to slumber may interrupt your sleep.

Pay Attention to Your Inner DJ

Finally, the optimum time to exercise is when it is convenient for you. Consider the following factors:

1. Your natural energy levels are as follows: Are you a morning person or a night person? Adjust your exercises to coincide with your peak energy cycles.

2. Your schedule: Can you set aside time in the morning, lunchtime, or evening? Choose a timetable that works in with your regular routine.

3. Your objectives: Are you looking to lose weight, gain energy, or reduce stress? Certain times of day may be more advantageous for achieving various goals.

4. Experiment and fine-tune: Don't be scared to experiment with different times to find out what works best for your body and mind. Adjust your workout plan based on how you feel before, during, and after your workouts.

Remember that consistency is essential. Choose a time that you can commit to on most days of the week, even if it is not your "ideal" time. The most essential thing is to begin moving and enjoy the numerous advantages of regular exercise.

So, ditch the tight schedules and accept your own rhythm. Find the time to move with delight, achieve your objectives, and appreciate the power of your unique body, whether you dance with the morning or chase the evening stars. After all, the greatest time to exercise is when you do it. Lace up your sneakers, crank up your inner music, and take on the clock one mindful movement at a time!

Where to Exercise

Forget about filthy treadmills and overcrowded gyms. Finding the proper spot to workout beyond 60 is about kindling delight, igniting motivation, and creating your own individual "fitness oasis." Imagine breaking free from the limits of habit and entering a world where movement combines perfectly with your interests, environment, and personal rhythm.

The entire planet is your gym! Let's look at some fascinating alternatives to the regular gym:

1.   **Nature's Symphony:** Surrender to the exhilarating energy of the great outdoors. Walk or jog through a lush park, climb a gorgeous track, or do yoga on a sunny beach. The beauty of nature adds a calming aspect to your workout, improving mood and lowering stress.

2. **Aquatic Aquaventure:** Immerse yourself in the delightful realm of water. Water workouts are

low-impact, supportive, and very soothing, whether it's moderate aqua aerobics in a local pool, exhilarating laps in a lake, or simply floating serenely.

3. Rhythms of Community: Find delight in moving with others. Join a senior dancing class, a tai chi group in the park, or a zumba class at the community center. While training, socializing adds a layer of enjoyment and keeps you motivated.

4. Home Sweet Gym: Turn your living environment into a personal exercise oasis. For at-home training, invest in some resistance bands, yoga mats, or lightweight dumbbells. You may use online instructions, guided routines, or make your own personalized exercises.

5. Canvas Creative: Express yourself via movement! Consider dancing to your favorite music, enrolling in a chair yoga session that focuses on balance and flexibility, or gardening with attentive posture and stretches. Connecting activity to your interests improves both your workout and your attitude.

Identifying Your Oasis

Remember that the ideal "where" is less about geography and more about creating an atmosphere that inspires you and makes you happy. Consider the following suggestions:

1. Match your interests: Do you enjoy nature? Water? Music? Choose an activity that appeals to your interests.

2. Pay attention to your body: Choose low-impact workouts that are easy on your joints and appropriate for your fitness level.

3. Accept convenience: Choose a location that is convenient for you and meets your schedule.

4. Make it Social: Find a workout companion or a group to add a layer of fun and accountability.

5. Experiment and investigate: Do not be frightened to try new things! You may find hidden abilities and interests.

Proper Breathing Techniques

Building a strong core isn't just about crunches and sit-ups for seniors over 60; it's also about recognizing the power of your breath. Proper breathing methods, like a bellows, stimulate your core muscles, boost workout efficacy, and improve your general well-being. So, instead of taking short breaths, use these strategies to access the hidden weapon of core exercises:

1. Diaphragmatic Deep Dive: Instead of chest puffs, try belly breaths! Engage your diaphragm, the muscle behind your ribs, by allowing your belly to expand on inhalation and pull in on exhalation. This deep breathing method naturally activates your core muscles, offering stability and support during any workout.

2. Coordination is essential: Link your breath to your motions. Inhale to prepare for the effort, such as lowering yourself into a squat, and exhale to apply power, such as pushing yourself back up. This coordinated breathing increases muscular activation and reduces tension.

3. Find Your Rhythm: There is no such thing as a one-size-fits-all breathing rhythm. Experiment with various inhale-exhale ratios to find the one that works best for you. Short, controlled breaths may be beneficial for some workouts, while longer, deeper breaths may be required for others. Find your flow by listening to your body.

4. Take a deep breath: During exercise, holding your breath traps air and stresses your core. Even during difficult motions, remember to completely exhale. This maintains optimum oxygen flow to your muscles, avoiding dizziness and increasing the benefits of exercise.

5. Postural Perfection: Posture is important for breathing. Sit or stand tall, shoulders relaxed, spine extended. This allows your diaphragm to move freely, improving the efficacy of your breath and increasing core activation.

6. Mindful Exhales: Pay attention to your exhalations. Consider how each breath expels stress and tiredness. This focused technique not only increases core activation but also relieves tension and promotes relaxation, leaving you feeling revitalized after your workout.

7. Practice Makes Perfect: Just like any other skill, acquiring healthy breathing requires time and effort. Include diaphragmatic breathing in your regular routine, even if it is as easy as walking or cleaning. The more you focus on your breathing, the easier it will be to incorporate it into your core workouts.

Remember that correct breathing is about more than simply getting enough oxygen; it's about unleashing the power within you. By combining these strategies into your core exercises, you'll discover a new source of strength, increase the efficiency of your workouts, and develop a newfound connection to your body. Breathe deeply, move powerfully, and learn the transformational power of breath for a healthy, empowered core at any age!

More Than Just Motion

Remember that your "fitness oasis" is more than simply a location to workout; it's also a haven for your mental health. You may connect with nature, express yourself creatively, and form a supportive community here. It's where you move with enthusiasm, overcome obstacles, and appreciate the lively vigor you possess.

So, break free from tradition, explore the limitless options, and create your own "fitness oasis." Allow movement to serve as your artwork, your playground, and your celebration of living a vigorous life after 60. Accept the freedom to move, the thrill of discovery, and the strength of your own distinct beat. Begin exploring now to discover a world of movement that feels good, nourishes your spirit, and enables you to be your strongest, happiest self.

Chapter 2: Seated Core Exercises

Building a strong core does not involve expensive equipment or hard activity. Even when seated, you can work your core muscles, improve posture, and increase stability with these simple exercises:

1. Seated Cat-Cow

• Sit tall on a chair with your feet flat on the floor. Inhale while arching your back, sinking your tummy, and bringing your chin to your chest (cow position).
• Exhale while rounding your back, dropping your chin to your chest, and clenching your core (cat stance).
• Repeat 10-12 times, focusing on feeling your back muscles and core engage with each breath.

2. Seated Spinal Twists

• Sit tall, with your feet level on the floor and your hands on your thighs.
• Slowly twist your upper body to the right, gazing over your shoulder while maintaining your hips forward.
• Hold for 5 seconds, then gently twist back to the center.

• Repeat on the opposite side, aiming for 5-6 twists per side.

3. Seated Arm Circles

• Sit tall with your feet level on the floor and your arms at shoulder height stretched to the sides.
• Make little circles with your arms, first forward for 10-12 times, then backward for another 10-12 reps.
• Maintain proper posture by activating your core while moving your arms.

4. Seated Leg Lifts

• Sit tall, with your feet level on the floor and your hands lightly resting on your knees.
• Lift one leg off the floor slowly, keeping it straight and engaged.
• Hold for 3 seconds, then slowly lower it back down.
• Repeat with the second leg, aiming for 8-10 raises each leg.

5. Seated Pelvic Tilts

• Sit tall, with your feet level on the floor and your hands resting on your thighs.

• Press your lower back into the chair, then slowly tuck your pelvis beneath you, tightening your core and squeezing your glutes.
• Hold for 5 seconds, then gently return to neutral.
• Repeat 10-12 times, focusing on the contraction and relaxation of your core muscles.

6. Seated Side Bends

• Sit tall, with your feet level on the floor and your arms resting on your hips.
• Slowly bend your upper body to one side, bringing your hand to the floor while keeping your back straight.
• Hold for 5 seconds, then gently return to the center and repeat on the opposite side.
• Aim for 5-6 bends per side.

7. Seated March

• Sit tall, with your feet level on the floor and your hands resting on your knees.
• Bring one knee up to your chest, tapping your shin with your hand.
• Alternate legs swiftly, as if marching.
• Continue for 30-60 seconds, keeping your core engaged and your back straight.

8. Seated Chair Pose

• Sit tall on the edge of your chair, feet level on the floor, and hands on your thighs.

• Lift your heels slowly off the ground, utilizing your core and leg muscles.

• Hold for 10-15 seconds, then slowly drop your heels back down.

• Repeat 5-8 times, concentrating on keeping good posture throughout.

9. Seated Abdominal Crunches

• Sit tall, with your feet level on the floor and your arms folded over your chest.

• Lean forward slowly, rounding your back and using your core muscles.

• Hold for 3 seconds, then gently return to the upright posture.

• Repeat 8-10 times, focusing on the contraction and relaxation of your abdominal muscles.

10. Seated Deep Breathing

• Sit tall, with your feet flat on the floor and your hands softly resting on your tummy.

• Inhale deeply through your nose, feeling your tummy expand.

• Exhale gently through your lips, pulling your belly button in towards your spine.
• Continue for 5-10 minutes, concentrating on your breath and feeling your core muscles engage with each inhale and expiration.

Remember to listen to your body and alter workouts as required. Begin with simpler motions and progressively increase repetitions and sets as your strength and confidence grow. With constant practice, these sitting exercises can help strengthen your core, improve your posture, and raise your general well-being, leading to a happier and more active life beyond 60.

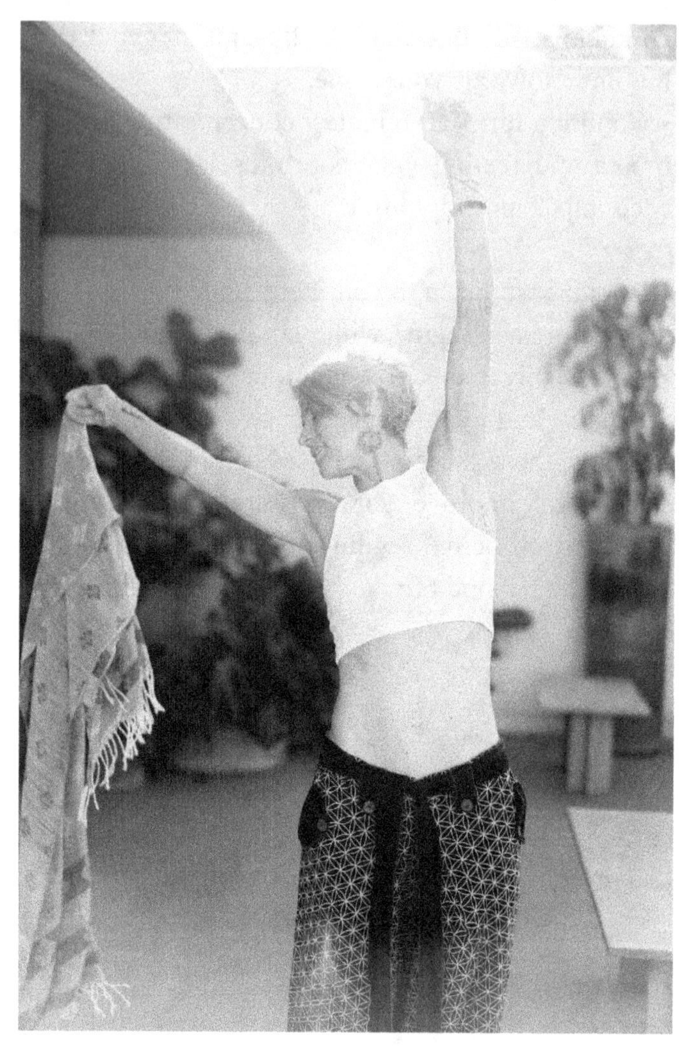

Chapter 3: Standing Core Exercises

1. Heel Raises

• Stand tall with your feet shoulder-width apart and your toes pointed forward.
• Lift your heels slowly off the ground, clench your calves, and hold for a second.
• Lower your heels and repeat 10-15 times.

2. Front Wall Presses

• Face a wall with your arms shoulder-width apart and your elbows bent at 90 degrees.
• Lean slightly forward and put your palms on the wall, as if pushing it away.
• Hold for 10 seconds, then release and repeat 10-12 times.

3. Bird-Dog

• Begin on all fours with hands under shoulders and knees under hips.
• Maintain a flat back and an engaged core.
• Extend one arm forward and the opposing leg back, maintaining both straight.

• Hold for a second, then return to the beginning position and repeat on the opposite side.
• Perform 8-10 repetitions per side.

4. Side plank

• Start on your side with your elbow directly under your shoulder and your legs stacked.
• Lift your hips off the ground, making a straight line from head to toe.
• Hold for 10-15 seconds, then swap sides and repeat.

5. March in Place

• Stand tall with your feet hip-width apart.
• Bring one leg up to your chest, then lower it back down.
• Rep with the other leg.
• Continue marching in place for 30 seconds to 1 minute.

6. Arm Circles

• Stand with your feet shoulder-width apart and your arms stretched out to the sides at shoulder height.
• Form tiny circles with your arms forward for 15-20 repetitions.

• Then switch direction and form circles backward for another 15-20 reps.

7. Chair Squats

• Stand in front of a solid chair with your feet shoulder-width apart.
• Slowly lower yourself as if sitting on a chair, maintaining your back straight and your core engaged.
• Don't sit all the way down; just get as low as you can comfortably.
• Push yourself back up to standing and repeat 10-12 times.

8. Balance Reaches

• Stand tall with your feet hip-width apart.
• Extend one arm straight out to the side, then gently stretch forward with the opposing hand while keeping your balance.
• Return to the starting position and repeat on the other side.
• Perform 8-10 repetitions per side.

9. Heel Taps

• Stand tall with your feet shoulder-width apart.
• Lift one leg slightly off the ground and tap your heel behind you while keeping your knee bent.

• Return to the starting position and repeat with the other leg.
• Perform 10-12 repetitions per side.

10. Walking Lunges

• Take a large stride forward with one leg, dropping your hips until both knees are bent at 90-degree angles.
• Return to the beginning position by pushing through your front heel, and then repeat with the opposite leg.
• Perform 8-10 repetitions per side.

Add diversity to your program by experimenting with other standing core exercises or altering the ones listed above to suit your fitness level. Remember to have fun and remain active!

Chapter 4: Mat Core Exercises

1. Seated Marching

• Sit on the mat with your back straight.
• Lift one leg toward your chest, then the other, in a marching motion.
• Maintain an erect posture throughout by using your core.

2. Pelvic Tilts

• Lie on your back with your legs bent and your feet flat.
• Tilt your pelvis upward, flattening your lower back into the mat.
• Hold for a time, then let go. Repeat.

3. Leg Raises

• Lie down on your back with your legs straight.
• Lift one leg a few inches above the ground, then drop it back down.
• Alter your legs, keeping your core engaged and your back pressed against the mat.

4. Seated Russian Twists

• Sit on the mat with your knees bent and your feet flat.
• Clasp your hands together and twist your body to one side, then the other.
• Engage your core and move in a controlled, rhythmic manner.

5. Bridge Exercise

• Lie on your back, knees bent and feet hip-width apart.
• Lift your hips toward the sky, forming a straight line from your shoulders to your knees.
• Squeeze your glutes and focus your core before lowering back down.

6. Modified Plank

• Begin on your hands and knees.
• Extend one leg back, then the other, preserving a straight line from head to heels.
• Hold for a few seconds, making sure your core is tight.

7. Knee-to-Chest Stretch

• Lie on your back and raise one knee to your chest, gripping it with your hands.

• Hold for 15-30 seconds, experiencing a mild stretch in your lower back.
• Rep with the other leg.

8. Side Leg Lifts

• Lie on one side with your legs straight.
• Lift the upper leg a few inches, then drop it back down.
• Keep your core engaged and your body in a straight line.

9. Cobra Stretch

• Lie on your stomach with your palms near your shoulders.
• Lift your chest off the mat while keeping your lower body planted.
• Hold for a few seconds, then drop back down.

10. Dead Bug Exercise

• Lie on your back with your arms stretched toward the ceiling and your legs elevated.
• Lower one arm and the opposing leg to the floor, then swap sides.
• Maintain control by keeping your lower back firmly against the mat.

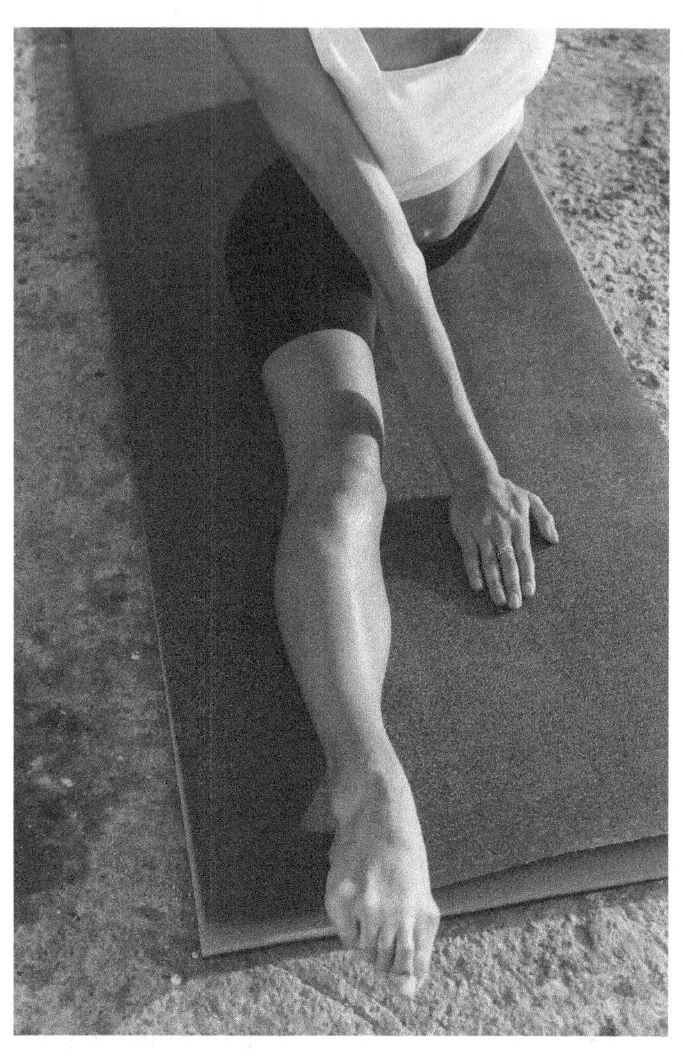

Chapter 5: Walking Core Exercises

Walking is a great form of exercise for seniors, but did you know you can also activate your core and improve your general health while strolling? Here are ten simple walking core exercises that can convert your daily stroll into a little strength session:

1. Heel Lifts

• Lift your heels off the ground for a few seconds after each stride as you walk.
• This works your calves and core muscles for increased stability.

2. Arm Swings

• Swing your arms lightly back and forth as you walk.
• Keeping proper posture and exercising your shoulder and core muscles.

3. Marching in Place

• While walking, lift one leg up to your chest as if marching.

• Alter your legs for a minute or two, maintaining your core engaged and your back straight.

4. Knee Lifts with a Twist

• Lift one knee and shift your upper body towards that knee as you walk.
• For a minute, alternate legs and twists, working your obliques and core.

5. Deep Belly Breathing

• Concentrate on your breathing while you walk.
• Inhale deeply through your nose, feeling your belly expand, then exhale gently through your mouth, bringing your belly button in.
• This engages your diaphragm and core muscles.

6. Pelvic Tilts

• Tuck your pelvis beneath you when walking, engaging your core and glutes.
• Hold for a few seconds, then return to neutral.
• Repeat numerous times throughout your stroll.

7. Shoulder Shrugs

• Raise your shoulders towards your ears for a few seconds while walking, then relax them.

• Repeat this shrug-and-relax action for a minute, activating your upper back and core muscles.

8. Side Arm Reaches

• As you walk, raise one arm out to the side at shoulder height, working your side waist muscles.
• Hold for a few seconds, then draw your arm back and repeat on the opposite side.

9. Walking Backwards

• Walk a short distance while gazing over your shoulder.
• This tests your balance and core stability, keeping you awake and engaged.

10. Stair Steps

• If you come across stairs, take one step at a time.
• Focus on controlled movements and using your core muscles to raise your weight with each step.

These basic actions can improve your core strength, posture, and general well-being, making your regular stroll even more useful and fun. So, lace up your sneakers, engage your core, and transform your next stroll into a strength session! Every step contributes toward a healthier, happier self.

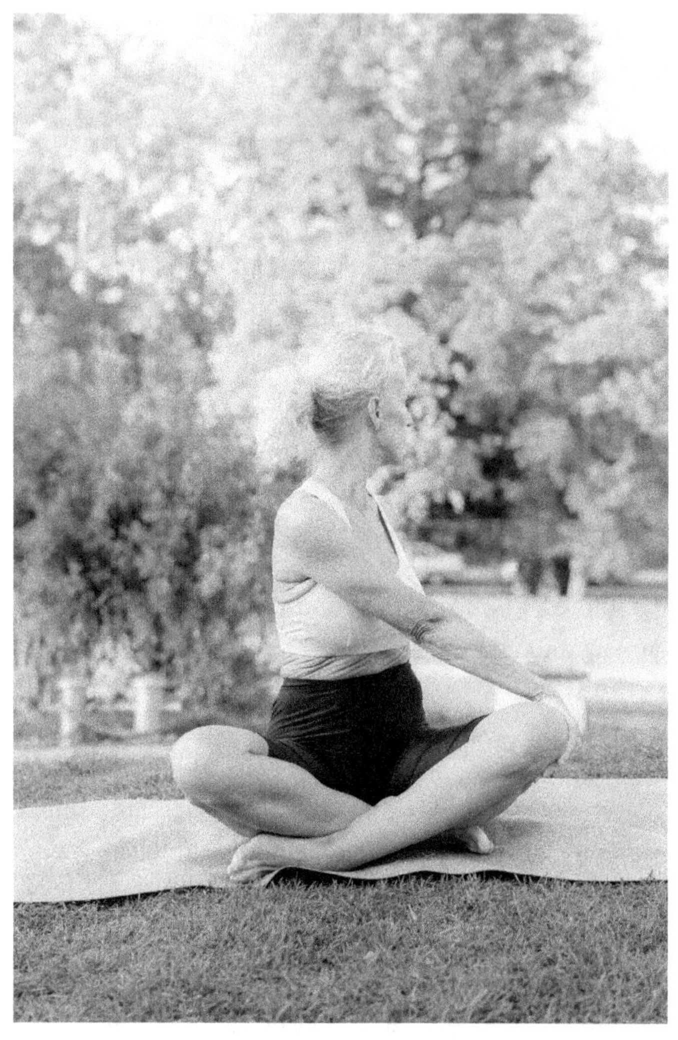

Chapter 6: Partners Exercises

Exercising with a partner may be a great way to remain motivated, have fun, and add a social element to your fitness regimen. Here are some mild and effective activities for seniors over 60 to do with a partner:

1. Seated Pass the Ball

• Face each other and stretch your legs comfortably. Hold a soft ball between you.
• Pass the ball back and forth with precise motions, activating your core and arm muscles.
• Begin gently and progressively raise the speed for a fun challenge.

2. Standing Balance Challenge

• Stand facing each other, holding hands with arms outstretched.
• One person softly leans back, relying on the other for support.
• Hold for a few seconds, then trade roles.
• This builds core muscles and improves balance while also encouraging trust and communication.

3. Partner Arm Swings

• Stand side by side, facing the same direction, with hands connected overhead.
• Swing your arms in tandem forth and backward, activating your shoulders and core muscles.
• Coordination your motions and experience the excitement of dancing together.

4. Gentle Leg Presses

• Face each other and stretch your legs comfortably. Place your soles against each other's knees.
• Gently squeeze your knees toward each other for a few seconds, then release. Repeat 10-12 times.
• This develops leg muscles and improves core stability while providing a fun interaction.

5. Side-to-Side Lunges

• Hold hands while you stand side by side, facing the same direction.
• Take a lunge step to the side, one person at a time, while maintaining balanced postures.
• This builds leg muscles, improves coordination, and fosters collaboration.

6. Walking Circles

• Hold hands and create a tiny circle, facing each other.

• Begin by walking gently around the circle, gradually increasing your speed.

• Maintain proper posture and core engagement as you move together.

7. Balloon Volleyball

• Stand across from one other, each carrying a giant inflated balloon.

• Gently volley the balloon back and forth with your hands or forearms, working on control and synchronization.

• This is a fantastic method to train your core and upper body muscles while also adding a lighthearted aspect.

8. Chair Dips

• Sit facing each other on firm seats, hands on each other's knees.

• One person lowers down gently, while the other gives support by pressing back on their knees.

• After a few repetitions, switch positions and engage your core, arm, and leg muscles.

9. Partner Stretches

• Face each other and grab for each other's opposing arms or shoulders.

• Hold for a few seconds, experiencing the soft stretch in your upper back and core.

• This improves relaxation and develops your core posture.

10. Walking Meditation

• Walk side by side in quiet, focusing on your breath and coordinated steps.

• This mindful stroll enhances mental well-being while training your core muscles and balance.

Exercising with a partner may be a terrific way to inspire each other, keep accountable, and bring a new layer of delight to your fitness regimen. So, find a partner, choose your favorite routines, and get ready to move, laugh, and improve your health together!

Chapter 7: Exercises with Weights

Even beyond 60, adding modest weights to your exercise regimen may be a terrific method to increase strength, enhance bone density, and promote metabolism. Here are some beginner-friendly exercises that you may do with small dumbbells or weighted balls (about 2-5 lbs) to help you keep strong and active:

1. Bicep Curls

• Stand tall with your feet hip-width apart and a dumbbell in each hand, palms facing front.
• Bend your elbows and slowly raise the weights to your shoulders. Pause, then slowly drop them back down.
• Repeat 10-12 times, focusing on feeling your biceps engage.

2. Tricep Extensions

• Stand tall with your feet hip-width apart and a dumbbell in each hand overhead, palms facing front.
• Bend your elbows and drop the weights behind your head, keeping your upper arms near to your ears.

• Pause, then gently return your arms to the beginning position.
• Repeat 10-12 times, focusing on feeling your triceps engage.

3. Shoulder Presses

• Stand tall with your feet hip-width apart, gripping a dumbbell in each hand at shoulder height with your hands facing front.
• Slowly raise the weights straight up overhead until your arms are completely stretched.
• Pause, then slowly lower them back to shoulder height.
• Repeat 10-12 times, focusing on feeling your shoulders engage.

4. Lateral Raises

• Stand tall with your feet hip-width apart and a dumbbell in each hand at your sides, palms facing down.
• Raise your arms out to the sides slowly until they are parallel to the floor.
• Pause, then slowly drop them back to your sides.
• Repeat 10-12 times, focusing on feeling your side shoulders engage.

5. Front Raises

• Stand tall with your feet hip-width apart and a dumbbell in each hand at your sides, palms facing inward.

• Raise your arms straight out in front of you until they are parallel to the floor.

• Pause, then slowly drop them back to your sides.

• Repeat 10-12 times, focusing on feeling your front shoulders engage.

6. Bent-Over Rows

• Stand tall with your feet hip-width apart and a dumbbell in each hand, palms facing back.

• Hinge at your hips and gently bend your knees while maintaining your back straight.

• Pull the weights up to your chest, pressing your shoulder blades together.

• Pause, then slowly drop them back down.

• Repeat 10-12 times, focusing on feeling your back muscles engage.

7. Leg Presses

• Sit in a chair with your feet flat on the floor and a dumbbell on each knee.

• Press your feet into the floor, lengthening your legs slightly.

- Pause, then gradually return to the starting position.
- Repeat 10-12 times, focusing on feeling your quadriceps engage.

8. Overhead Tricep Dips

- Hold onto a solid chair or counter with your hands shoulder-width apart.
- Step your feet back, maintaining your body in a straight line.
- Slowly bend your elbows, lowering your body to the floor until your elbows are 90 degrees bent.
- Pause, then push yourself back up to the starting position.
- Repeat 5-8 times, focusing on feeling your triceps engage.

9. Chair Squats

- Place your feet hip-width apart in front of a strong chair.
- To maintain balance, extend your arms straight out in front of you.
- Slowly lower your body as if sitting on a chair, maintaining your back straight and your core engaged.
- Pause at the bottom, then push yourself back up to the starting position.

• Repeat 10-12 times, focusing on feeling your leg muscles activate.

10. Weighted Walk

• Hold a light dumbbell in each hand while you walk around your house or at a park.
• Maintain proper posture and use your core muscles while you walk.
• Continue for 10-15 minutes, progressively increasing the length as you gain strength.

Remember to utilize weights that are comfortable for you and to listen to your body. Begin with less weight and progressively add more as you gain confidence. It is more vital to focus on perfect form and controlled motions than on lifting huge weights. Including these light weight workouts in your program will significantly improve your strength, balance, and general well-being. So, take your weights, accept the challenge, and discover the strength you possess!

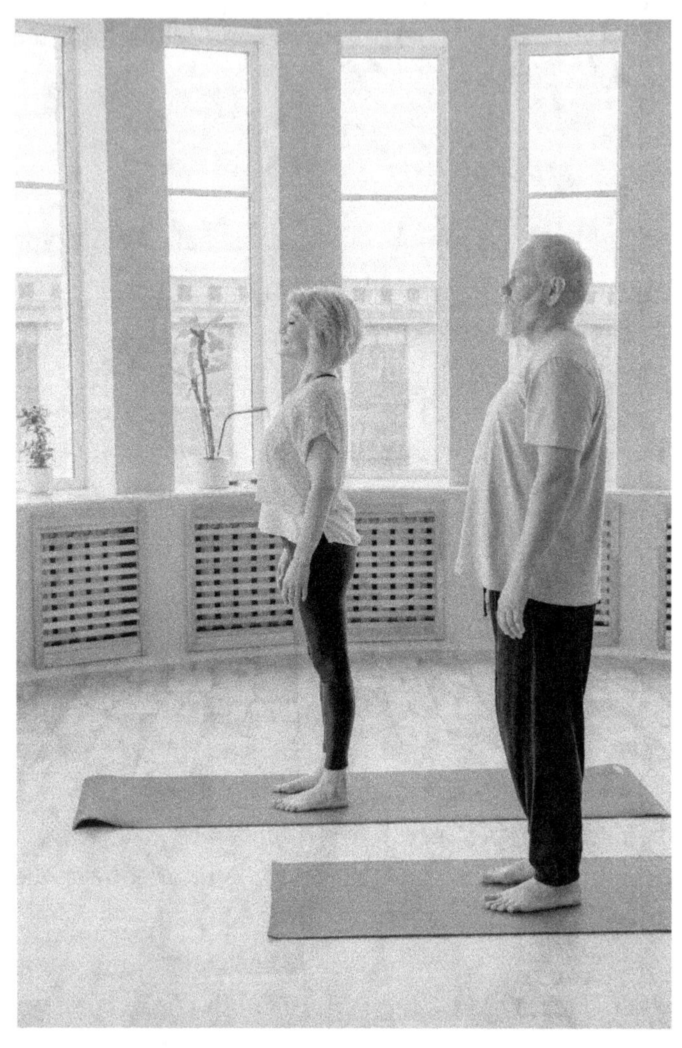

Chapter 8: Exercises for Ache and Pain Relieve

Living with aches and pains doesn't have to limit your mobility! Gentle exercise can be an effective tool for easing stiffness, improving flexibility, and lowering discomfort in seniors over the age of 60. Here are some safe and effective activities to help you get relief:

1. Neck Rolls

• Sit or stand tall, shoulders relaxed.
• Roll your head in a circular motion five times clockwise and five times counterclockwise.
• Repeat 2-3 times more.

2. Shoulder Shrugs

• Sit or stand tall, shoulders relaxed.
• Lift your shoulders gently towards your ears, hold for a few seconds, and then slowly release.
• Repeat 10-12 times.

3. Arm Circles

• Sit or stand tall, arms outstretched to the sides at shoulder height.

- Make little circles with your arms, forward for 10-12 times.
- Then backward for another 10-12 reps.
- Keep your core engaged.

4. Gentle Leg Swings

- Sit in a chair with your feet flat on the floor.
- Swing one leg forth and backward slowly, keeping your leg straight and relaxed.
- Rep with the other leg.
- Continue for 5-10 swings per leg.

5. Seated Knee Lifts

- Sit in a chair with your feet flat on the floor.
- Lift one knee slowly towards your chest, hold for a few seconds, then gently lower it back down.
- Rep with the other leg.
- Continue with 8-10 lifts per leg.

6. Ankle Circles

- Sit or stand tall with your feet flat on the floor.
- Make five clockwise and five counterclockwise circles with your ankles.
- Repeat 2-3 times more.

7. Deep Breathing

• Close your eyes and take a comfortable seat or lie down.

• Inhale deeply through your nose, feeling your tummy expand.

• Exhale gently through your lips, bringing your belly button in.

• Continue for 5-10 minutes, concentrating on your breath and feeling your body relax.

These easy exercises are an excellent approach to begin introducing movement into your life while relieving aches and injuries. Remember that even modest motions may make a great impact in your comfort and general well-being. So, keep moving, listen to your body, and enjoy the path to a more active and pain-free life!

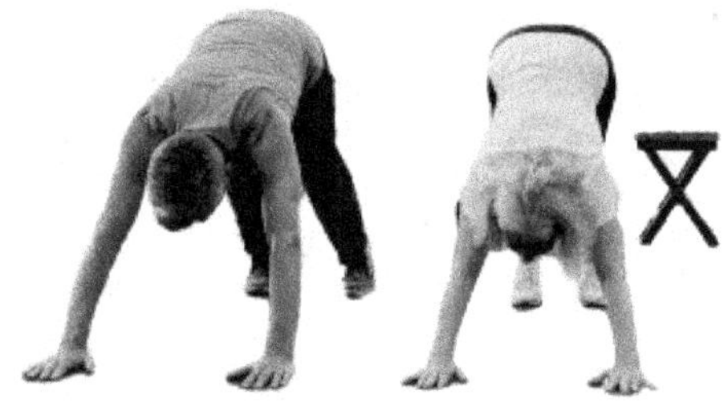

Chapter 9: Nutrition Tips for Core Health

Building a strong core requires more than just crunches and sit-ups; it also requires fuelling your body with the correct nourishment. Your core muscles thrive on a balanced diet rich in certain nutrients, just as a robust structure requires a good foundation. So, put down the protein bars and fatty takeout and dig into these basic health dietary suggestions that will have you standing tall and feeling powerful from the inside out:

1. Join the Fiber Force:

Consume 25-35 grams of fiber each day from fruits, vegetables, whole grains, and legumes. Fiber keeps you full, assists digestion, and even promotes your gut microbiota, which supports fundamental health indirectly. Think apples, berries, leafy greens, brown grains, oats, lentils, and beans for a healthy core.

2. Join the Lean Protein Squad:

Instead of high-fat meats, go for lean protein sources such as chicken breast, fish, tofu, and almonds. Protein is the fundamental building block of all muscles, including your core. To ensure your core receives the building blocks it needs to be strong and robust, aim for 0.8 grams of protein per kilogram of body weight every day.

3. Don't Be Afraid of Healthy Fats:

Not all fats are the same! Substitute unsaturated fats found in avocados, olive oil, nuts, and seeds with saturated fats found in processed meals. These fats not only replenish your core muscles, but they also help with inflammation and general wellness.

4. Hydrate for Harmony:

Water is essential for all physical functions, including your core. To keep your muscles hydrated and working properly, drink eight to ten glasses of water every day. Remember that even minor dehydration can have an impact on your core strength and performance.

5. Avoid Sugar Saboteurs:

Refined sugars and sugary beverages are enemies of core wellness. They raise your blood sugar, cause inflammation, and drain your vitality, leaving you lethargic and limiting your workout efforts. Reduce your intake of sugary snacks and processed meals, and replace them with natural sweeteners such as fruits and honey in moderation.

6. Spice Up Your Life:

Anti-inflammatory spices like ginger, turmeric, and cayenne pepper might help lessen core pain and stiffness, especially after exercises. So, don't be scared to try new things and give a gourmet touch to your meals while pampering your core.

7. Pay Attention to Your Body:

Because no two bodies are alike, pay attention to your hunger and satiety signs. Don't overeat, but don't miss meals either. A well-balanced and consistent diet ensures that your core receives the nutrients it requires throughout the day to be strong and function well.

Keep in mind that good core strength is developed from within. By concentrating on these nutrition guidelines, you'll be laying the groundwork for maximum core health, leaving you feeling motivated, energized, and ready to face any obstacle life throws your way. So, eat well, exercise regularly, and let your core shine!

Importance of a Balanced Diet

Consider your body to be a great orchestra, with each organ representing a brilliant musician weaving together a symphony of life. Our health is dependent on a harmonic combination of nutrients - a balanced diet - just as this concert requires every instrument to play its role. But why is this equilibrium so important? Let's explore the melody of wonderful food:

1. The Macronutrient Melody:

Consider carbohydrates, proteins, and lipids to be the core chords of your health. Carbohydrates provide energy, proteins help build and repair tissues, while fats keep you full and help your brain work. Each is important, but an unbalanced symphony, dominated by sugary snacks or fatty pleasures, will result in a discordant melody from your body.

2. Vitamin and mineral harmony:

These micronutrients are the subtle accents that elevate the tune. Vitamin A for eyesight, iron for oxygen transport, and calcium for strong bones all contribute to the health symphony. Failure to hit any of these crucial notes might result in off-key performances, such as weariness, brittle hair, or reduced immunity.

3. Fiber's Rhythm:

Fiber operates like a continuous drumbeat, keeping your digestive system in sync. It improves intestinal health, decreases cholesterol, and even controls blood sugar levels. Constipation, bloating, and even an increased risk of chronic illnesses might result from skipping this vital pulse.

4. The Water Dance:

Picture a parched orchestra, with instruments breaking and melodies fading. This is what occurs when water, the key conductor of biological functions, is ignored. Dehydration throws the entire system out of sync, whereas hydrated cells correlate to bright health.

5. Variety in Composition:

True musical expertise is found in diversity. A healthy diet, similarly, thrives on diversity. Accept the vibrant colors of fruits and vegetables, the earthy tones of whole grains, and the rich notes of proteins from many sources. This nutrient-dense symphony feeds your body while delighting your taste buds.

6. The Harmony of Moderation:
Overplaying can ruin even the most exquisite melody. Overeating in any food type, even healthy ones, can throw the balance off. The key to a harmonic performance is moderation, which ensures you experience the entire symphony of nutrients without any unpleasant discords.

Keep in mind that a balanced diet is a dance of deliberate decisions, not a strict rulebook. Pay attention to your body's desires, try new flavors, and emphasize nutrient-rich selections. When you approach food as a symphony for your health, you will not only fuel your body but also nurture a lively melody of health that will resound throughout your life. So, pick up your fork, eat mindfully, and let your body perform the lovely symphony of excellent health!

Foods that Support Core Strength

Forget about crunches and sit-ups! Building a strong core after 60 starts at the grocery store, not the gym. Choosing the appropriate meals feeds your muscles, protects your bones, and improves your general well-being, laying the groundwork for a strong core and an active lifestyle. So, instead of sugary cereals and processed snacks, fill your shopping cart with these core-strengthening powerhouses:

1. Leafy Green Champions:

Spinach, kale, and collard greens are core health champions. They include calcium, magnesium, and vitamin K, which help to strengthen your bones, enhance flexibility, and prevent osteoporosis, all of which are important for a healthy and supported core. For a nutrient-dense boost, add them to salads, smoothies, or even soups.

2. Lean Protein Partners:

Chicken breast, fish, tofu, and lentils aren't just for athletes! These lean protein sources provide the building blocks for strong core muscles. Aim for 0.8 grams of protein per kilogram of body weight every day to ensure your core gets the amino acids it needs to be strong and robust.

3. Fiber Fantastic Four:

Beans, berries, sweet potatoes, and whole grains are your stomach's greatest friends, and a happy gut equals a happy core! Fiber controls digestion, decreases inflammation, and keeps you feeling full, improving energy levels for those training sessions.

From substantial lentil soups to sweet potato fries, embrace their varied textures and flavors.

4. Vitamin C Crusaders:

Citrus fruits, bell peppers, and broccoli are high in vitamin C, which is necessary for collagen formation. Collagen keeps your connective tissues strong and flexible, supporting your core muscles and encouraging general joint health. Squeeze some sunshine into your day with a morning grapefruit or add bright bell peppers to your stir-fry for a vibrant core boost.

5. Water Warriors:

Never underestimate the strength of simple old water! Dehydration may sap your vitality and weaken your muscles, jeopardizing your core strength. Aim for eight to ten glasses of water every day to maintain your body hydrated and working properly, allowing your core to operate at its best.

6. Spice Up Your Life:

Turmeric, ginger, and cayenne pepper aren't simply taste enhancers; they also have anti-inflammatory effects that can help lessen core pain and stiffness, especially after exercises. Sprinkle turmeric on your roasted vegetables, add ginger to your morning smoothie, or add a dab of cayenne pepper to your soup for a spicy and health-promoting touch.

7. Mindful Munching:

Ditch the late-night chips and sugary sweets. Choose healthful snacks such as almonds, seeds, yogurt with berries, or apple slices with almond butter. These deliver long-lasting energy, satisfy cravings, and keep your core nourished throughout the day.

A strong core is not formed overnight. It's a journey fuelled by the intentional decisions you make every day at the store and in your kitchen. By choosing these core-loving foods, you'll be creating the groundwork for a healthy, active lifestyle that will leave you feeling powerful and ready to meet any obstacle life throws your way. So, take your grocery list, enjoy the symphony of tastes, and let your core sing the tune of power and well-being!

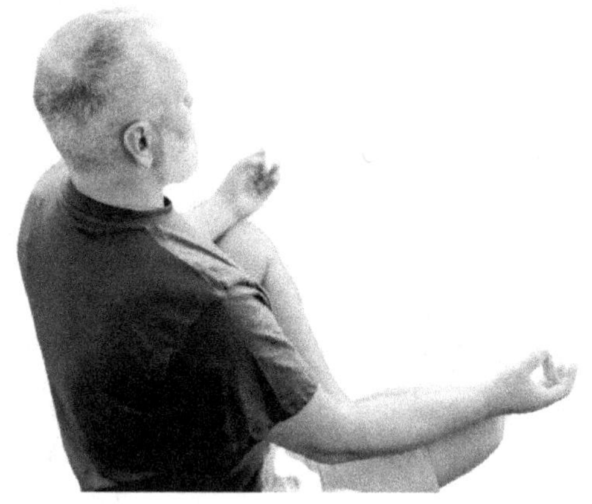

Conclusion

As you finish this book, a gratifying resonance stays inside you - a song of fresh power sung by your core's awakened muscles. This voyage inside your physical symphony has been a trip of discovery, not only of chiseled abs and toned torsos, but also of a profound resilience woven into the very fabric of your existence.

You have constructed a fortress of stability with each breath and each regulated movement, a foundation that allows you to traverse the world with greater confidence. The days of anxiety on the stairs and the constraints imposed by a weak core are long gone. You now rise to face each obstacle, your stride solid and sure, your back straight, a mute witness to the inner strength that is blooming.

However, this empowerment goes well beyond the physical sphere. You've discovered a source of energy, a vitality that reignites the joy of movement, the excitement of discovery, and the freedom to embrace life with open arms. Whether it's the joy of chasing your grandkids across the park, the exciting rhythm of a fast stroll with friends, or the peaceful serenity of maintaining your garden, your core hums with a fresh power that magnifies every sensation.

A song of confidence plays a perfect counterpart to this symphony of athletic skill. It glows in your eyes as you confront new difficulties, in your unflinching drive as you conquer barriers. It is confidence that allows you to move beyond of your comfort zone, to embrace the unknown, and to create your own masterpiece on life's canvas.

Be rest assured that age is not a conductor who determines the pace of your life. You are the conductor, in command of your inner strength, renewed vitality, and unshakeable confidence. You have silenced the naysayers both inside and beyond, demonstrating that the human spirit can blossom at any age, that a strong core is more than simply carved lines, but the unwavering song of resilience it plays.

Allow the reverberation of these activities to reverberate throughout you. Carry the power you've earned in your motions, but also in your very soul. Walk tall, breathe deeply, and let the world see the vivid symphony your center is now conducting. This isn't simply the end of a book; it's the start of a victorious return to your own bodily symphony - a masterpiece in the making, crafted by the strength of your robust core.

Go forth, conquer your world, and never cease finding the strength that is within your core. The adventures await!

Workout Planner

My workout planner

DATE

DAY	ACTIVITIES	TIME	REMARK
DAY:1			
DAY:2			
DAY:3			
DAY:4			
DAY:5			
DAY:6			

NOTES

My workout planner

DAY	ACTIVITIES	TIME	REMARK
DAY:1			
DAY:2			
DAY:3			
DAY:4			
DAY:5			
DAY:6			

NOTES

My workout planner

DATE

DAY	ACTIVITIES	TIME	REMARK
DAY:1			
DAY:2			
DAY:3			
DAY:4			
DAY:5			
DAY:6			

NOTES

My workout planner

DATE

DAY	ACTIVITIES	TIME	REMARK
DAY:1			
DAY:2			
DAY:3			
DAY:4			
DAY:5			
DAY:6			

NOTES

My workout planner

<table>
<tr><td>DATE</td></tr>
</table>

DAY	ACTIVITIES	TIME	REMARK
DAY:1			
DAY:2			
DAY:3			
DAY:4			
DAY:5			
DAY:6			

<table>
<tr><td>NOTES</td></tr>
</table>

My workout planner

| DATE | |

DAY	ACTIVITIES	TIME	REMARK
DAY:1			
DAY:2			
DAY:3			
DAY:4			
DAY:5			
DAY:6			

| NOTES |